Descartes and Newton: Pioneers of Modern Philosophy and Science

Most of the content is based on and inspired by a video performed to the young historian **Carlos Blanco**

Most of the content is based on and inspired by a video of an interview with the young historian Carlos Blanco. And it was translated and adapted into a book created by

JOSE MOYA

with the purpose of scaling the importance of higher academic training

ISBN: 9798854587686

DEDICATION

To those who seek knowledge and delve into the pages of history with curiosity and passion. To the tireless dreamers and lovers of science and philosophy, who find inspiration in the brilliant minds of the past to forge a better future.
This book is dedicated to Carlos Blanco, whose passion for sharing the legacy of great minds has opened the doors to new horizons of knowledge. Thank you for your tireless work and for guiding us through the intricacies of human thought.
It is also dedicated to all those who, like Descartes, Newton, and Einstein, challenge the limits of knowledge and relentlessly pursue the truth. May this book be a celebration of their legacy and an invitation to continue exploring the mysteries of the universe and human nature? May the flame of knowledge always burn in our hearts, and may each page of this book inspire us to question, reflect, and grow.
With gratitude and admiration,
Jose Moya

Descartes, Newton and Einstein

CONTENT

Descartes, Newton and Einstein

ACKNOWLEDGMENTS

I want to express my most sincere gratitude to all the people who contributed to the creation of this book. Without their support, dedication, and enthusiasm, this project would not have been possible.

First and foremost, I thank Carlos Blanco Pérez, whose story and passion for knowledge inspired every page of this work. Thank you for sharing your knowledge and being an endless source of motivation.

I also want to extend my gratitude to all the researchers, authors, and scholars whose works and studies on the topics of this book have provided us with a solid and enriching foundation. Their contributions have been invaluable in shaping this work.

Special thanks go to AMAZON, GOOGLE, LLM OpenAI, and others, for providing us with the tools and resources that allowed us to carry out this project efficiently and effectively.

Likewise, I want to thank my friends and family for their unwavering support throughout the entire process of creating this book. Their words of encouragement and moral support were an invaluable boost to keep going.

Finally, my deepest appreciation goes to all those readers who venture to explore these pages. I

sincerely hope that you find in this book a source
of learning, inspiration, and reflection.
With gratitude,
Jose Moya

BOOK INTRODUCTION:

The purpose of this book is to encourage everyone to be interested in knowledge. When you learn enough, you can intertwine expressions that can arouse curiosity in others and motivate them to learn more. When you discover that others want to listen to you and perceive the benefits of attracting attention, then you will seek the best information to nourish your thoughts, improve your beliefs, and influence us to become better individuals. You never know where the new flame of learning will arise and the advantages that we will all have by becoming providers of the best content on social networks.

This book delves into the lives and contributions of two exceptional figures who shaped the course of modern philosophy and science: René Descartes and Sir Isaac Newton.

Throughout these pages, we explore their groundbreaking ideas, their struggles, and the profound impact they left on the world.

Descartes, the brilliant French philosopher, is famously known for his axiom "Cogito, Ergo Sum" - "I think, therefore I am." We will trace his journey from childhood to his immersion in the Jesuit school, where he delved into classical languages, mathematics, and philosophy. Descartes' quest for certainty led him to doubt everything, including his own existence, in his methodical "Discourse on the Method." We will uncover his ontological argument for God's existence and the controversies surrounding his philosophical inquiries.

In contrast, we encounter Sir Isaac Newton, the enigmatic English scientist, who revolutionized our understanding of the universe. We will explore his upbringing and education, where his extraordinary talent for mathematics shone. Newton's famous encounter with an apple tree is the stuff of legends, but his contributions extend far beyond that moment. We will delve into his groundbreaking discoveries in optics, mathematics, and monumental work on the universal law of gravitation.

Both Descartes and Newton faced challenges

and opposition during their lifetimes, but their legacies still endure. We will examine the influence of their ideas on contemporary thought and how their contributions laid the foundations for modern scientific inquiry and philosophical exploration.

Join us on this captivating journey through the lives and minds of these exceptional individuals as we unravel the stories of Descartes and Newton and their lasting impact on the world.

The vast majority of the content of this book and the inspiration comes from enjoying a video about the television program Crónicas Marcianas 1999, where they interview a young Spanish prodigy, named Carlos Blancos, at a very young age, delights us with his advanced academic training derived from his precocious intellectual gifts and I assume the great effort of him and his parents by inducing him to read history from his first years of life. When listening to the pleasant story, available only in the important Spanish language, pleasant, however, interrupted by the interlocutor, and with multiple repeated phrases, language fillers typical of a good conversation, I understood that materials with such good content should be published in the English language because it is the most spoken language in the world and in a format for reading because there are still regular readers who will appreciate it. That said, all the credit that emanates from my effort to write this work goes to Carlos Blanco and his bibliography is available at the following link:

https://bit.ly/carlos-blanco

In good time, Carlos Blanco, thank you very much, and congratulations on your great contribution.

In addition, I must emphasize that for the writing and translation, use the benefits that chatGPT 4.0 offers us, which for me is exceptional because it puts the commas and periods where they should go and writes what you dictate or reports in an impressive way.

I must also add that any minimum or higher monetary income that this book generates is to self-finance the publishing costs, for spending time and resources on transcriptions, revisions, development, conversion of audio to text, applications, etc. But above all, to add useful content for everyone on the great information highway that is the Internet.

If Carlos Blancos, who deserves all the credits, feels alluded to or offended or uncomfortable or used for being the one chosen to escalate his career in a different language, in my superior opinion, and/or the conversion of the format from casual audio to professional writing and/or does not consider the effort and/or my resources as a writer, doctor, humanist beneficial to his legacy, not only do I apologize in advance and publicly. I am also willing to abandon any story related to him. Despite the fact that I will ask your permission to distribute it and despite the fact that you have answered it in the affirmative or have not answered it in the negative.

I report that I am not for profit, my profession as a free-practice doctor supports me and not that of a writer and my interest is none other than to scale brilliant minds to the highest possible level so that humanity knows the benefits of exceptional academic training.

CHAPTER 1: INTRODUCTION TO RENÉ DESCARTES: THE PHILOSOPHER WHO COINED "COGITO, ERGO SUM"

René Descartes, a French philosopher born in 1596 in La Haye, Turin (now France), belonged to a family of the lower nobility. Descartes received an intensive education, entering the Jesuit College of La Flèche at the age of eight, where he studied a wide range of subjects, including classical languages, mathematics, and philosophy. His studies exposed him to the scholastic practice of aligning human reason with Catholic doctrine.

At the age of 16, Descartes left the Jesuit school and pursued law, but he never practiced as an attorney. Instead, he enlisted in the army of Prince Maurice of Orange, where he spent his time pondering philosophical and scientific questions rather than military affairs. Descartes had a particular aversion to cold temperatures, attributed to pneumonia he contracted due to extreme cold.

Descartes' life took a significant turn when he embarked on a pilgrimage to Italy and later settled in Holland in 1628, where his remarkable scientific career began. In 1637, he published his famous work, "Discourse on the Method," challenging conventional wisdom and traditional beliefs. In this work, Descartes employed his method of doubt to question everything, including his own existence. This led him to formulate his famous phrase, "Cogito, Ergo Sum" - "I think, therefore I am." Descartes described the thinking thing, "res cogitans," as a conception that understands, affirms, denies, wants, imagines and feels.

Descartes also explored the existence of God through an ontological argument based on the idea of a perfect, infinite being. His work laid the foundation for modern philosophy and earned him the title of the "founder of modern philosophy."

Join us in the following chapters as we delve deeper into the life and ideas of René Descartes, unraveling the fascinating journey of this remarkable philosopher.

CHAPTER 2: THE CHILDHOOD AND EARLY EDUCATION OF RENÉ DESCARTES

René Descartes was born on March 31, 1596, in La Haye, a small town in Turin, France. He came from a family of the lower nobility, which granted him certain privileges and opportunities for his education. From an early age, Descartes showed signs of mental sharpness and intellectual curiosity, paving the way for his brilliant future as a philosopher and scientist.

In his youth, Descartes received a high-quality education. At the age of eight, he entered the prestigious Jesuit College of La Flèche, located in Anjou, France. In this educational institution, he immersed himself in a wide range of disciplines, including classical languages, mathematics, and philosophy. The Jesuits, known for their focus on education and scholarship, significantly influenced Descartes' intellectual formation.

It was at La Flèche College where Descartes had his first contact with mathematics and geometry, which sparked a profound interest in him. During his time at the school, Descartes also delved into philosophy, exploring the works of classical and medieval philosophers, as well as the teachings of Christian theologians.

René Descartes is attributed to his famous phrase: "Ahí donde fueres, haz lo que vieres" ("Wherever you go, do what you see"). However, this expression is strongly influenced by the Jesuit spirit of the time, which advocated for remaining always open to new theories and discoveries, and for acquiring all the knowledge possible.

This phrase, "Ahí donde fueres, haz lo que vieres," reflects Descartes' attitude towards learning and acquiring knowledge. He himself embraced this philosophy and applied it to his life and work. Descartes stood out for his unceasing desire to seek the truth and his willingness to accept new ideas and concepts, which led him to develop a rigorous and revolutionary philosophical and scientific method.

However, not everything was easy for

Descartes on his academic journey. Despite having a keen mind and a thirst for knowledge, he also faced personal and health challenges. His time at the Jesuit college coincided with a period of convalescence due to pneumonia he contracted because of extreme weather conditions, hence his aversion to cold and meditating until 11 in the morning before getting out of bed.

Throughout his life, Descartes was always open to new perspectives and constantly in search of the truth. His legacy is not only found in his contributions to philosophy and science but also in his progressive approach and willingness to question established beliefs.

Despite the difficulties, Descartes demonstrated tenacity and a passion for learning that led him to excel in his studies. His education at the Jesuit college laid the foundations for his future intellectual career, and it was there that his rigorous and methodical approach to knowledge and research began to take shape.

The next chapter will take us to know Descartes' transition from education to adulthood, his travels and explorations, and how these events shaped his unique philosophical and scientific perspective.

CHAPTER 3: DESCARTES' JOURNEY TO
SELF-DOUBT AND PHILOSOPHICAL
EXPLORATION

The brilliant philosopher René Descartes embarked on a unique intellectual journey that led him to question everything and explore philosophy from its foundations. In his work "Discourse on the Method," Descartes presents his famous method of doubt, a powerful tool for examining the truthfulness of all beliefs and knowledge.

In this journey of self-discovery, Descartes faced uncertainty and skepticism, questioning everything he had learned and assumed until then. Through methodical doubt, Descartes sought to attain firm and true knowledge, discarding any idea that could be questionable or doubtful.

At a crucial moment in his meditation,

Descartes came to the conclusion that he could be deceived by a powerful evil genius pushing him to believe in falsehoods. This radical hypothesis of universal doubt led him to question even the most apparent truths.

However, Descartes found one indubitable certainty: the fact that he was doubting implied that he was thinking, and the act of thinking confirmed his existence as a thinking being. Thus, his famous assertion emerged: "Cogito, ergo sum" - "I think, therefore I am."

With this solid foundation of his own existence as a thinker, Descartes could begin to reconstruct his system of knowledge from scratch. From this certainty, he developed his philosophy based on the idea that thought and reason are the fundamental sources of knowledge.

Descartes also explored the relationship between the mind and the body, arguing that the mind and body are distinct substances but interact in the union of a person. This dualistic conception of the mind and body became a central theme in his philosophical investigations.

Throughout his life, Descartes continued to explore and develop his ideas, leaving a lasting legacy in philosophy and science. His method of doubt and his celebrated assertion "Cogito, ergo sum" remain landmarks in philosophical thought and the quest for truth.

In the following chapters, we will delve deeper into René Descartes' additional achievements and contributions, as well as the challenges and controversies he faced in his unrelenting pursuit of truth and knowledge.

CHAPTER 4: THE REVOLUTIONARY "DISCOURSE ON THE METHOD" BY DESCARTES

Descartes' "Discourse on the Method" is a groundbreaking work that marked a turning point in the history of philosophy and science. Published in 1637, this work is presented as a treatise in which Descartes lays out his method of doubt and his systematic approach to attaining true knowledge.

In this work, Descartes begins with a powerful declaration of intent, expressing his desire to free his mind from all preconceived ideas and to accept only those that can withstand the most rigorous scrutiny. His method of doubt consists of questioning any belief or knowledge that may be subject to doubt or error.

Descartes starts his doubt with information perceived through the senses, arguing that the senses can deceive us and, therefore, are not a reliable source of knowledge. He then extends his doubt to the ideas and notions he has acquired throughout his life, questioning whether some of them may have been influenced by external opinions or erroneous ideas.

The ultimate goal of Descartes' doubt is to arrive at indubitable certainty, a solid starting point from which he can reconstruct his system of knowledge. It is at this point that he reaches the famous assertion: "Cogito, ergo sum" - "I think, therefore I am." This certainty becomes the foundation upon which he builds his philosophy.

From this certainty, Descartes advances in his reasoning and concludes that God exists as an innate reality in the human mind and that the existence of God is essential to guarantee the truthfulness of human knowledge. This idea is part of his ontological argument for the existence of God.

The "Discourse on the Method" also addresses scientific and mathematical questions. Descartes presents analytical geometry as a powerful tool for solving geometric problems through the use of coordinates. His rigorous and mathematical approach significantly influenced the development of science.

This work had a profound impact on the philosophy and science of its time, and its legacy endures to this day. The method of doubt and the assertion "Cogito, ergo sum" continue to be fundamental elements in the quest for truth and knowledge.

In the following chapters, we will explore more deeply the philosophical and scientific contributions of René Descartes, as well as the criticisms and controversies that his ideas generated in his time and in posterity.

CHAPTER 5: DESCARTES' ONTOLOGICAL ARGUMENT FOR THE EXISTENCE OF GOD

One of the most prominent aspects of Descartes' philosophical thought is his ontological argument for the existence of God. This argument is presented in his work "Discourse on the Method" and is based on the idea of a perfect and infinite being.

Descartes starts from the premise that he has an innate idea of a perfect being, that is, a being that possesses all possible perfections. The notion of a perfect being is so clear and distinct in his mind that it cannot be a product of his own invention or experience. Descartes argues that if he, as a finite and imperfect being, has the idea of a perfect being, then there must exist a real and supreme being that possesses all those perfections.

Descartes' ontological argument can be summarized in the following steps:

We have the innate idea of a perfect and infinite being.

A perfect and infinite being possesses the perfection of existing both in the mind and in reality.

If it only existed in the mind and not in reality, it would not be a perfect being, as a being that exists both in the mind and in reality would be more perfect than one that only exists in the mind.

Therefore, a perfect and infinite being must exist both in the mind and in reality.

Descartes considers existence to be perfection. A being that exists is more perfect than one that does not exist. If a perfect being only existed in the mind and not in reality, then it would not be truly perfect, as existing, in reality, is a higher characteristic than existing only in the mind.

Therefore, Descartes concludes that the perfect and infinite being, whom he calls God, exists both in the human mind and in reality. God is the cause of the innate idea of perfection in Descartes' mind, and His existence is necessary to guarantee the truth and certainty of human knowledge.

Descartes' ontological argument has been the subject of numerous debates and criticisms throughout the history of philosophy. Some philosophers have questioned the validity of assuming that existence is perfection, while others have argued that the argument does not provide conclusive proof of God's existence.

The ontological argument defends the existence of God based on the idea that there is a perfect and infinite being, which is God, and that this superior being must exist in reality and not just in our minds. We, as finite and imperfect beings, cannot be the cause of the existence of a perfect being, as the most perfect cannot derive from the less perfect, which would lead to a contradiction.

If we imagine all possible qualities and perfections, they must have their origin in some being that contains them all. If I had created myself, I would have given myself all the qualities I can conceive. However, by recognizing that I am a finite and imperfect being, I deduce that these perfect qualities must come from a superior being, which has created them by itself, that is, God. The idea of God as a perfect being must have been placed in me by this superior being, and therefore, God must exist.

Another famous ontological argument related to being is as follows: when we think of concepts like a mountain, the inseparable concept of a valley is also involved. However, thinking about the existence of a mountain is not the same as affirming that a mountain exists. On the contrary, when thinking about God, the idea of existence is inseparable from the idea of God, as a perfect being must necessarily exist to be truly perfect. Thus, the existence of God is derived.

This ontological argument has received various criticisms, including that of Pierre Gassendi, a contemporary of Descartes. Gassendi argued that existence is not a property that can be proven, which was precisely what Descartes was trying to demonstrate, so this type of argument may not be valid. Despite the criticisms, Descartes' ontological argument has been the subject of debate and reflection throughout the history of philosophy.

Despite the criticisms, Descartes' ontological argument remains a relevant and discussed topic in philosophy and theology, leaving an indelible mark on the history of human thought.

CHAPTER 6: CRITICISMS AND CONTROVERSIES SURROUNDING DESCARTES' IDEAS

Descartes' philosophical thought has not been exempt from criticisms and controversies throughout history. While his ideas have been influential and revolutionary, they have also sparked debates and challenges from other philosophers and thinkers.

One of the main criticisms directed at Descartes is his ontological argument for the existence of God. Many philosophers have objected that having an innate idea of a perfect being does not necessarily imply that such a being exists in reality. They argue that existence is not a necessary characteristic for perfection and that the idea of a perfect being could simply be a construction of the human mind.

Furthermore, some critics have pointed out that the notion of "perfection" is subjective and depends on each individual's conceptions. What one considers perfect may not be so for another, undermining the validity of Descartes' ontological argument.

Another significant criticism of Descartes' ideas comes from empiricist philosophy, which emphasizes the importance of experience and the senses as fundamental sources of knowledge. Empiricists argue that Descartes' method of doubt, which questions all knowledge acquired through the senses, leads to radical skepticism and undermines the foundation of science and empirical research.

Regarding Cartesian dualism, which posits a separation between the mind and the body, some philosophers have objected that this raises issues about how these two distinct substances interact. The mind-body interaction has been the subject of debates and has led to alternative theories seeking a more integrated view of human nature.

Additionally, Descartes has also been criticized for his conceptions about the role of animals in nature. By considering animals as mere machines without mind or soul, Descartes has been subject to criticisms from advocates of animal rights and animal ethics.

Despite these criticisms and controversies, Descartes' legacy in philosophy and science remains significant. His ideas and methods of reasoning have influenced the way we conceive knowledge and reality. Although some of his ideas have been challenged, his contribution to human thought is undeniable and continues to be studied and reflected upon to this day.

CHAPTER 7: SIR ISAAC NEWTON: A COMPLEX AND BRILLIANT MIND

Sir Isaac Newton was a scientific genius whose legacy left an indelible mark on the history of science. Born on January 4, 1642, in Woolsthorpe Manor, England, Newton was an extraordinary individual, and his mind was filled with complexities and talent.

From a young age, Newton showed great interest and skill in mathematics and the sciences. At the age of 17, he entered the famous University of Cambridge to study philosophy, which at that time included mathematics, physics, chemistry, and other scientific disciplines.

During his time at Cambridge, Newton lived through a period of great creativity and discovery. At a crucial moment in his life, while he was away from the university due to a plague epidemic, he developed his revolutionary ideas about gravity. The famous law of universal gravitation, which explains how objects attract each other, was one of his most outstanding achievements and forever changed our understanding of the universe.

In addition to his contributions to the field of physics, Newton also made important advances in mathematics. He was one of the pioneers in the development of infinitesimal calculus, a powerful mathematical tool used to solve problems in physics and other areas of science.

Newton's personality was complex. He was known for his reserved nature and reluctance to immediately publish his discoveries, which sometimes led to conflicts with other scientists of his time. However, when he finally published his research, it was received with great admiration and respect by the scientific community.

Despite his brilliance, Newton was also a controversial figure. He had a strained relationship with some of his contemporaries and was occasionally embroiled in disputes and controversies over the authorship of certain ideas and discoveries.

In addition to his legacy in science, Newton was also a person with interests in alchemy, theology, and mysticism. While some have argued that these areas of interest did not influence his scientific achievements, others believe that his holistic approach to knowledge contributed to his genius and unique worldview.

Sir Isaac Newton passed away on March 20, 1727, in London, leaving behind an extraordinary legacy that has endured through the centuries. His complex and brilliant mind continues to be a source of inspiration for scientists and thinkers worldwide, and his work continues to be studied and celebrated as one of the foundational pillars of modern science.

CHAPTER 8: NEWTON'S FORMATIVE YEARS AND HIS ENCOUNTER WITH THE APPLE

The early years of Newton's life were marked by his curiosity and passion for knowledge. He was born on January 4, 1642, in Woolsthorpe Manor, England, into a modest family. From a young age, he showed great interest in nature and mathematics, which led him to explore various subjects on his own.

At the age of 17, Newton entered the University of Cambridge to study philosophy. During his time at the university, he excelled in his exceptional ability to solve mathematical problems and conduct scientific research. However, his student years were interrupted by the plague epidemic that struck England.

During this time, Newton returned to his home at Woolsthorpe Manor and embarked on a period of intense reflection and research. It was during this time of confinement and isolation that the famous encounter with the apple occurred.

Legend has it that while Newton was sitting under an apple tree, an apple fell and hit his head. This event led him to ponder the nature of the force that caused the apple to fall toward the Earth. This reflection was the starting point of his investigations into the law of universal gravitation.

The law of universal gravitation, which Newton developed later in his life, states that all objects in the universe attract each other with a force proportional to their masses and inversely proportional to the square of the distance that separates them. This groundbreaking law explained for the first time how celestial bodies, such as the Moon and the planets, move and maintain their orbits around the Sun.

The encounter with the apple is an iconic symbol of Newton's curiosity and intuition, as well as his focus on the scientific method and logical reasoning. Through his genius and perseverance, Newton managed to change our understanding of the universe and laid the foundations of modern physics.

Newton's formative years and his encounter with the apple are an example of how passion for knowledge and curiosity can lead to great scientific discoveries. His legacy endures to this day and continues to inspire generations of scientists and thinkers in their quest to understand the universe that surrounds us.

CHAPTER 9: NEWTON'S INNOVATIVE DISCOVERIES IN OPTICS AND MATHEMATICS

Sir Isaac Newton made revolutionary discoveries in two fundamental fields: optics and mathematics. These contributions marked a turning point in science and continue to be fundamental pillars in their respective disciplines.

Optics:

In the field of optics, Newton conducted experiments and research on the nature of light. His most notable work in this area was his famous experiment with a glass prism. Newton demonstrated that white light from the sun is composed of a variety of colors, leading to the discovery of the color spectrum. He documented this finding in his work "Opticks," published in 1704.

Furthermore, Newton also formulated the theory that light is composed of particles, which conflicted with the prevailing theory at that time, which held that light was a wave. His corpuscular theory of light influenced the later development of wave theory and laid the groundwork for the theory of wave-particle duality in modern physics.

Mathematics:

In the field of mathematics, Newton made pioneering contributions to the development of infinitesimal calculus. Along with the German mathematician Gottfried Leibniz, Newton is considered one of the creators of modern calculus. Calculus is a powerful mathematical tool that allows the study of changes and rates of variation and has been fundamental in the development of physics and other sciences.

Newton formulated fundamental concepts in calculus, such as the fundamental theorem of calculus and the chain rule, which are essential in the study of functions and derivatives.

Moreover, his research in mathematics also encompassed topics such as the study of differential equations and the theory of infinite series.

Newton's discoveries in optics and mathematics transformed the way we understand the world and laid the groundwork for many subsequent scientific developments. His work continues to be studied and applied today, and his genius continues to inspire scientists and mathematicians in their quest to understand the fundamental laws that govern the universe.

CHAPTER 10: THE UNIVERSAL LAW OF GRAVITATION: NEWTON'S MAGNUM OPUS

The universal law of gravitation is considered Sir Isaac Newton's masterpiece and one of the most remarkable achievements in the history of science. This revolutionary law explained how bodies attract each other throughout the universe and laid the foundations for modern physics.

Formulation of the Law:

Newton presented his theory of universal gravitation in his work "Philosophiæ Naturalis Principia Mathematica" ("Principia" for short), first published in 1687. In this book, Newton formulated the three laws of motion, known as Newton's laws, and developed his theory of gravitational force.

According to the law of universal gravitation, any two bodies in the universe attract each other with a force proportional to the product of their masses and inversely proportional to the square of the distance between them. This gravitational force acts along the straight line that joins the centers of the two bodies.

Explanation of Celestial Motion:

The law of universal gravitation was crucial in explaining the motion of celestial bodies in the solar system. Newton demonstrated that the gravitational force between the Sun and the planets is what keeps the planets in their orbits around the Sun.

Furthermore, Newton applied his law of gravitation to the Moon and showed that it is the gravitational force between the Earth and the Moon that causes the ocean tides.

Enduring Impact:

The publication of the "Principia" changed the way scientists understood the world and paved the way for the development of modern physics. The law of universal gravitation provided a precise mathematical explanation for the motion of celestial bodies and allowed for accurate predictions about their orbits and movements.

The legacy of the law of universal gravitation continues to be relevant today. Its influence extends beyond physics and has been crucial in space exploration and astronomical navigation.

Sir Isaac Newton left an indelible impact on science with his masterpiece, the law of universal gravitation. His genius and ability to understand and explain the fundamental laws of the universe continue to be a source of inspiration for generations of scientists and thinkers in their quest to understand the cosmos.

CHAPTER 11: THE CHALLENGES AND TRIUMPHS OF NEWTON AS PRESIDENT OF THE ROYAL SOCIETY

Sir Isaac Newton was elected President of the Royal Society of London in 1703, a position he held for numerous years. During his time as president, Newton faced significant challenges and also achieved important triumphs in his leadership of this prestigious scientific institution.

Challenges as President:

One of the main challenges that Newton faced as president was dealing with politics and diplomacy within the Royal Society. The society was composed of scientists and scholars with different viewpoints and scientific approaches, which sometimes led to tensions and disputes among the members.

Furthermore, Newton was known for his reserved nature and often preferred to work in solitude rather than engaging in public debates and discussions. This sometimes drew criticism from other members who expected greater participation and public leadership from their president.

Triumphs as President:

Despite the challenges, Newton achieved significant triumphs during his presidency. It was during his time as president of the Royal Society that he published his work "Opticks" in 1704. In this book, Newton presented his research on the nature of light and color, as well as his corpuscular theory of light.

Additionally, under his leadership, the Royal Society continued to foster scientific research and the exchange of knowledge among its members. The society became an important center of learning and experimentation, attracting scientists from across Europe.

Newton's Legacy in the Royal Society:

Newton's legacy as president of the Royal Society is still remembered and celebrated in the history of science. During his tenure, his leadership and scientific genius left a lasting mark on the institution and the scientific community at large.

His focus on rigorous scientific research and his emphasis on experimentation and the scientific method have left an indelible impact on the way science is conducted today.

Newton's time as president of the Royal Society was a period of challenges and triumphs, and his legacy continues to inspire future generations of scientists and thinkers to pursue the quest for knowledge and understanding of the world around us.

CHAPTER 12: NEWTON'S BATTLES WITH THE INSTITUTION AND HIS RELIGIOUS BELIEFS

Throughout his life, Sir Isaac Newton faced challenges and conflicts with the institution, and he also held religious beliefs that generated debates and controversies.

Battles with the Institution:

Newton had friction with the scientific community of his time due to his reserved nature and reluctance to share his research immediately. His meticulous approach to work and his desire for perfection made him cautious about publishing his discoveries. This generated criticism and discontent among other scientists who expected a more open exchange of knowledge.

Additionally, Newton faced disputes and conflicts with other scientists, such as the German mathematician Gottfried Leibniz, over who had invented infinitesimal calculus. These disputes, known as the "Calculus Controversy," led to tensions and rivalries between the two scientists and their followers.

Lai Lis accused Newton of plagiarizing his infinitesimal calculus. However, further investigations have revealed that both of them independently and in parallel arrived at the same conclusion. Lai Lis conducted his research in Germany without knowing that Newton was working on similar topics in England. The truth is that neither of them copied each other's ideas.

Newton, known for being resentful, gained recognition for his discovery of the decomposition of the seven colors of the rainbow through a prism. This achievement in optics and mathematics earned him the presidency of the prestigious Royal Society of London.

Once in office, Newton made a questionable decision. He commissioned a report on the matter with Lai Lis and forged his signature on the document. He formed an investigation committee, and the report stated that Lai Lis had plagiarized his ideas. As the president, his conclusions prevailed, but in reality, they were wrong because neither of them had plagiarized the other.

Religious Beliefs:

Newton had strong religious beliefs and dedicated much of his life to studying theology and alchemy. Although he is primarily known for his scientific contributions, he also wrote extensively on theological and biblical topics.

Newton was a Christian and believed in a God who created the universe. However, his theological views often differed from the predominant religious beliefs of his time. For example, Newton rejected the doctrine of the Trinity and the idea of the Holy Trinity, which generated controversy among religious leaders of the time.

His Legacy:

Despite the challenges and controversies, Newton's legacy in science and religion endures to this day. His contributions to physics and mathematics have been fundamental in the development of modern science, and his focus on the scientific method continues to be an inspiration for scientists around the world.

Regarding his religious beliefs, Newton considered himself a devout believer, and his interest in theology and alchemy shows his quest to understand the world and its relationship with the divine.

Ultimately, Newton's legacy encompasses both his scientific discoveries and his religious beliefs, reflecting the complexity and depth of his brilliant mind.

CHAPTER 13: THE LEGACY OF DESCARTES AND NEWTON IN MODERN SCIENCE AND PHILOSOPHY

The legacies of René Descartes and Isaac Newton in modern science and philosophy have left a profound mark on human thought and our understanding of the world. Their ideas and discoveries have been fundamental in the development of modern science and philosophy, and their influence remains relevant to this day.

Descartes and the Cartesian Method:

René Descartes is known for his rational approach and his philosophical method, known as the "Cartesian method." His emphasis on methodical doubt and deductive reasoning laid the foundation for modern scientific thinking.

The slogan "Cogito, ergo sum" ("I think, therefore I am") has become a cornerstone of Western philosophy and highlights the importance of thought as an undeniable certainty.

Furthermore, Descartes made significant contributions to analytic geometry and the theory of coordinates, laying the groundwork for the further development of geometry and algebra.

Newton and Classical Physics:

On the other hand, Isaac Newton is considered one of the most influential scientists of all time. His laws of motion and law of universal gravitation revolutionized our understanding of the universe and laid the foundation for classical physics.

The law of universal gravitation explained how bodies attract each other through invisible forces, and his rigorous mathematical approach allowed for precise predictions about the motion of planets and other celestial bodies.

Newton's scientific approach, based on observation, experimentation, and mathematical method, has been essential in modern science and has influenced the development of physics, astronomy, and other scientific disciplines.

Their Lasting Impact:

The legacy of Descartes and Newton continues to be relevant in modern science and philosophy. Their methods and approaches have inspired generations of scientists and philosophers to continue exploring the world and seeking answers to fundamental questions about the nature of the universe and ourselves.

Modern science and philosophy continue to be shaped by the foundations established by Descartes and Newton, and their legacy endures in the relentless pursuit of knowledge and understanding.

The significance of Descartes and Newton in modern science and philosophy is a testament to the magnitude of their contributions and the eternal relevance of their thinking in the quest for truth and understanding of the universe.

CHAPTER 14: THE LASTING INFLUENCE OF THEIR IDEAS ON CONTEMPORARY THOUGHT

The ideas of René Descartes and Isaac Newton continue to exert a profound influence on contemporary thought. Their philosophical and scientific approaches have left an indelible mark on various areas of knowledge and remain relevant to this day.

Descartes and Modern Philosophy:

Descartes' Cartesian method, based on deductive reasoning and methodical doubt, has served as a model for contemporary philosophical and scientific thinking. His emphasis on reason as the primary source of knowledge remains a central feature of modern philosophy.

Furthermore, Descartes was a pioneer in the idea that the mind and body are separate entities, influencing the later development of the philosophy of mind and psychology.

Newton and Modern Science:

Newton's laws of motion and the law of universal gravitation laid the foundation for classical physics and continue to be fundamental in modern science. His principles of conservation of energy and inertia have been applied in countless fields of physics and engineering.

Newtonian mechanics remains an invaluable tool for understanding the behavior of moving bodies, from everyday objects to space exploration.

Influence on the Philosophy of Science:

Both Descartes and Newton have influenced the contemporary philosophy of science. Their approaches to the scientific method and the relationship between theory and observation have been studied and debated in the philosophy of science.

The quest for truth and rational understanding

of the world, present in the ideas of Descartes and Newton, remain central themes in the study of epistemology and the philosophy of mind.

In Popular Culture:

The ideas of Descartes and Newton have transcended the academic sphere and permeated popular culture. Their quotes and concepts, such as Descartes' "I think, therefore I am" and Newton's law of universal gravitation, can be found in books, movies, and popular speeches.

The impact of their ideas is also reflected in modern technology and the development of science fiction, where concepts about the mind, time, and space find their roots in the works of these two great thinkers.

The Enduring Legacy:

The influence of Descartes and Newton on contemporary thought is a testament to the enduring nature of their ideas and the ongoing relevance of their contributions. Their legacy remains alive in the pursuit of knowledge, the quest for truth, and the effort to understand the complexity of the universe and ourselves.

As we move into the 21st century, the intellectual heritage of Descartes and Newton continues to inspire scientists, philosophers, and

thinkers to look to the future with an open mind
and an inquisitive spirit, in search of new ideas
and discoveries that enrich our understanding of
the world.

CHAPTER 15: THE UNPARALLELED CONTRIBUTIONS OF DESCARTES AND NEWTON

René Descartes and Isaac Newton, two intellectual giants of history, have left an unparalleled legacy in science and philosophy. Their contributions revolutionized human thinking and marked a turning point in the development of knowledge and understanding of the universe.

Descartes, with his Cartesian method and search for indubitable truth, laid the foundation for rational thinking and the modern scientific method. His emphasis on reason and the mind as sources of knowledge served as a beacon that illuminated the path toward rigorous scientific research and the pursuit of objective truth.

On the other hand, Newton, with his laws of motion and law of universal gravitation, revealed the invisible forces that govern the behavior of the universe. His mathematical approach and principles of conservation and equilibrium became the cornerstone of classical physics and the basis for the further development of science.

Both thinkers went beyond the established boundaries of their predecessors and challenged the prevailing beliefs of their time. Their brilliant and audacious minds marked a before and after in the progress of human knowledge and forever changed our understanding of the world.

The legacy of Descartes and Newton extends to the present day, and their influence endures in contemporary science and philosophy. Their ideas continue to inspire generations of scientists, philosophers, and thinkers to explore new frontiers and seek answers to fundamental questions about the nature of reality and the human being.

In summary, the unparalleled contributions of Descartes and Newton are a perennial reminder of the power of the human mind to unravel the mysteries of the universe and the unyielding drive of humanity for knowledge and understanding. Their legacy will endure as a

beacon of wisdom and an inexhaustible source
of inspiration for future generations.

53

CHAPTER 16: ALBERT EINSTEIN: A COMPLEX AND BRILLIANT GENIUS

Albert Einstein, one of the most prodigious minds in history, continues to be a subject of admiration and debate. When compared to Newton, the question arises: Who has been more relevant to science? Newton or Einstein? Both have left indelible marks on human knowledge, but Einstein's genius stands out for his abstract approach and astonishing theories.

From a young age, Einstein demonstrated an astonishing ability for self-directed learning. Despite limited education, at the age of 12, he already knew Euclidean geometry and showed signs of an incipient genius. His inquisitive mind and passion for the violin made him stand out as a peculiar and unique individual.

The pinnacle of his career came with his theory of relativity. In 1905, he published the special theory of relativity, which was based on the previous work of other scientists but carried his brilliant signature. However, it was in 1916 when he published his general theory of relativity, a masterpiece that completely reformulated our understanding of space and time.

According to Einstein's theory, bodies can deform space and time, leading to astonishing phenomena. The famous image of billiard balls deforming a rubber sheet illustrates how massive objects, such as planets and stars, curve space around them. Furthermore, his theory of general relativity introduced the idea that time is relative and can vary depending on the observer's frame of reference.

Einstein's theory challenged traditional conceptions and directly confronted Newton's well-established and proven theories. However, Einstein's genius lay precisely in his ability to refute what seemed logical and demonstrate the truth of his own theories through astronomical phenomena, such as the famous 1919 eclipse.

But his path was not without controversies and difficulties. At a time when no one believed in his ideas, he had to face skepticism and disbelief from other prominent scientists. Even after his theory was experimentally confirmed, some scientists resisted accepting his revolutionary approach.

Einstein also revealed himself to be a deeply religious man, a Zionist Jew who believed in an orderly and harmonious God. His famous phrase "God does not play dice with the universe" reflected his belief that everything has an explanation and underlying order.

Throughout his life, Einstein remained steadfast in his pacifist ideals and advocated for nuclear disarmament. He was deeply affected when his theories contributed to the development of the atomic bomb and regretted his role in advancing military technology.

Despite fame and worldwide recognition, Einstein always maintained his simplicity and sense of humor. Photographs of him sticking his tongue out have become symbols of his unique and charismatic personality.

Albert Einstein visited various countries, including Spain, Argentina, and Uruguay, leaving an indelible mark on each place he visited. His legacy endures in modern science, philosophy, and culture, and his genius continues to be a source of inspiration for future generations.

ABOUT THE AUTHOR

Dr. José Moya is a renowned medical specialist in the treatment and management of Vitiligo. With over 35 years of experience in the field of medical sciences, Dr. Moya has been distinguished for his innovative approach and dedication to helping people prevent and manage this skin condition.

Born in Bayamo, Cuba, Dr. Moya began his medical training in institutes that offered a comprehensive range of specialties, allowing him to acquire comprehensive and multidisciplinary knowledge.

But as I mentioned in the introduction of this book, it's not only about the life and work of these great characters but also a recognition and a special look at Carlos Blanco, a young Spanish man passionate about history and dedicated to sharing his knowledge through videos on Youtube. His ability to memorize and summarize numerous books he has read during his academic preparation has allowed Carlos Blanco to bring these topics to a wider audience through his videos

See more references about Carlos Blanco:
https://bit.ly/carlos-blanco

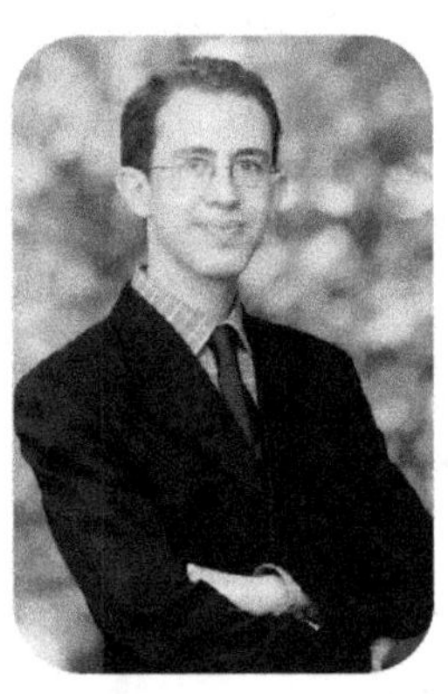

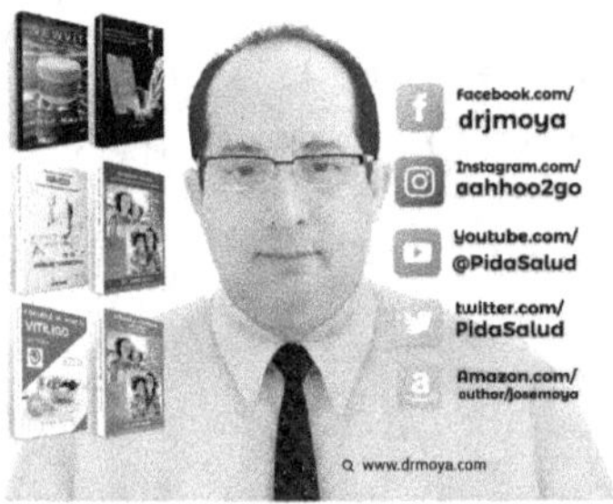

Visita:

www.amazon.com/author/josemoya

www.drmoya.com

www.ingramcontent.com/pod-product-compliance
Lightning Source LLC
Chambersburg PA
CBHW071058260726
48661CB00006B/2336